The Veteran's Toolkit for PTSD

The Veteran's Toolkit for PTSD

✦

Twenty Practical Ways to Successfully Cope with Post Traumatic Stress Disorder

Chaplain Ramsey Coutta, PhD

iUniverse, Inc.
New York   Bloomington

The Veteran's Toolkit for PTSD
Twenty Practical Ways to Successfully Cope with Post Traumatic Stress Disorder

The views expressed in this work are solely those of the author and do not necessarily reflect the views of the publisher, and the publisher hereby disclaims any responsibility for them.

iUniverse books may be ordered through booksellers or by contacting:

iUniverse
1663 Liberty Drive
Bloomington, IN 47403
www.iuniverse.com
1-800-Authors (1-800-288-4677)

Because of the dynamic nature of the Internet, any Web addresses or links contained in this book may have changed since publication and may no longer be valid.

ISBN: 978-1-4401-9858-8 (sc)
ISBN: 978-1-4401-9859-5 (ebk)

Printed in the United States of America

iUniverse rev. date: 01/04/2010

Contents

Hyperarousal

Introduction

This book is written for you the military veteran, whether you served in the Army, Navy, Air Force or Marines. It is for both the veteran who has been diagnosed with Post Traumatic Stress Disorder (PTSD), and the veteran who has not received a diagnosis but who is experiencing symptoms of PTSD. It is a toolkit, if you will, of twenty practical ways for the veteran to better cope with symptoms of PTSD. Most of these tools can be practiced alone to improve coping. This was done purposefully because there are many veterans who will never seek professional treatment, but who would like to learn some skills to improve their management of PTSD symptoms. However, there are a few tools in this book that it is recommended that a professional counselor, friend, chaplain or other close person be present to help guide and support the veteran. In these instances, the need for these other helpers is indicated as that tool is being described.

Post Traumatic Stress Disorder is divided into three primary clusters dealing with re-experiencing symptoms, avoidance symptoms and hyperarousal symptoms. Accordingly, this book is divided into these three main sections. The tools in each section are designed to specifically address symptoms that are found in each cluster. For example, flashbacks are considered a re-experiencing symptom, so there is a tool that addresses flashbacks in the re-experiencing section. You will also find a number of stories throughout this book to help illustrate what the symptoms of PTSD might look like in the life of a veteran. All of the stories are inspired by real life events experienced by veterans. However, each story is a mixture of different experiences by different veterans along with inspired details to better bring the story to life. All of the names are fictitious in order to protect the identities of those who experienced these traumatic events. If you find the stories too emotionally difficult, you can skip them and just read the material covering the tools. If in going through this book, you find your symptoms of PTSD starting to worsen significantly before they get better, you should seek out a helper such as a professional counselor, chaplain or go to a hospital emergency room, Vet Center, VA hospital, sick call, or seek someone higher up in you chain of command.

Most of the tools in this book need to be practiced several times to gain the most benefit. We rarely become skillful at something unless we practice it more than once. You may also want to spend more time with those tools that specifically relate to the symptoms you are experiencing. For example, if you are having trouble with panic attacks, then you will want to spend more time practicing the skills described in the tool on coping with panic attacks in the section on hyperarousal.

You should be aware that there is debate in the helping community as to whether PTSD or the symptoms of PTSD can be completely cured or simply managed. From my experience, a veteran's memories will always remain regarding his or her traumatic experiences. The symptoms of PTSD are typically worse in the early years after the traumatic event. However, as time passes and distance is put between the person and the events, they generally become better at managing their symptoms and the intensity of the symptoms tend to lessen. This book is based on the idea that the veteran should strive toward managing their symptoms, and the tools in this book are designed to support that goal.

Re-experiencing

Overwhelmed

PFC Stuart joined the Army and the airborne corp in a surge of patriotism after the attacks on 911. After finishing his training, his unit was sent to Iraq where they were responsible for patrolling a number of small villages around a large northern city. He patrolled in Humvees and on foot. He lost several friends to IED's and small arms attacks, and even on base after patrol insurgents regularly lobbed mortars and rockets on to it. While other soldiers in the unit became angry and vengeful after an attack, Stuart refused to join in their tactics of firing indiscriminately at unidentified targets. Their anger then turned on him as they accused him of sympathizing with the enemy.

Matters got worse when PFC Stuart watched one day as his best friend was in a Humvee as a turret gunner. The Humvee driver swerved to avoid colliding with an Iraqi truck, and the Humvee overturned crushing his friend. Stuart helped to recover the remains and even loaded the casket on the plane for the trip home. Shortly after this, his own Humvee was hit by an IED injuring no one, but leaving both him and the driver with concussions and recurrent headaches.

After he returned to the states, anxiety, depression and mood swings started to afflict him and he sought medical treatment. He was put on medication, but the improvement was minimal. In remembrance of the friends he lost, he had several tattoos put on both arms with the first name of each. A few months later, his unit was put on notice that they would be deployed again, this time to Afghanistan. During this time, his anxiety, depression, dreams and flashbacks started to worsen.

Once in Afghanistan, he was placed on a team that was responsible for responding to attacks on their forward base. Whenever a mortar, rocket or small arms attack took place, he and his team headed out to track down the attackers. At first, they struggled to make contact with the enemy, but eventually became better at locating and eliminating the threat. While PFC Stuart still continued to refrain from shooting at unidentified targets, he nevertheless found himself shooting more and more at enemy that were positively identified. The number of enemy he killed during his Afghanistan tour mounted to nearly twenty. While he knew the enemy would kill him if given the chance, he still could not fully reconcile in his mind taking the life of another person.

Deciding not to reenlist after he had served his time, he returned home and took a restaurant job waiting tables and enrolled in the local university. The job wasn't going that well because he was impatient with the customers and what he felt were their inane requests. It didn't help that some of the patrons would question him about the tattoos on his arm, so he started wearing long sleeves and considered getting rid of the tattoos surgically. He also felt more irritable and at times angry. In one incident, a bartender at a local bar asked to see his identification. Leaning over the bar, he growled angrily, "I've killed more men than you can count on two hands, so if I can kill I can drink!" He then stormed out of the bar while his friends looked on bewildered.

When someone would come to the door of his apartment, such as the pizza man, he would stand behind the door to gain tactical superiority. In class and with schoolwork he struggled to concentrate, as his thoughts and memories continued to return to his lost friends and combat experiences. Sleep was also elusive and this contributed to his constant depressed mood. At times he even thought about suicide, reasoning he would be free of his pain and reunited with those friends he lost. Fortunately, his girlfriend who had noticed his downward spiral, finally convinced him of the need to do something about his PTSD.

Tool 1

Learn About PTSD

Becoming educated and informed about the signs, symptoms and care for Post Traumatic Stress Disorder (PTSD) is one of the most effective ways to contribute positively to your recovery. When people have greater knowledge about something that is negatively affecting them, they feel more in control of it and its impact on their life. They are better able to identify what actions they can take to help themselves as well as knowing what actions are unhelpful and even destructive. Fear of the effects of PTSD on their life is lessened and they become more confident in their ability to live happily and productively.

PTSD is when a person experienced, witnessed or was confronted with an event where there was the threat of or actual death or serious injury. The event may have also involved a threat to the person's physical well-being or the physical well-being of another person. The person responded to the event with strong feelings of fear, helplessness or horror. The following are the seventeen symptoms of PTSD divided into three primary clusters of re-experiencing symptoms, avoidance symptoms, and hyperarousal symptoms.

Re-experiencing symptoms:
- Frequently having upsetting thought or memories about a traumatic event.
- Having recurrent nightmares.

- Acting or feeling as though the traumatic event were happening again, sometimes called a "flashback."
- Having strong feelings of distress when reminded of the traumatic event.
- Being physically responsive, such as experiencing a surge in your heart rate or sweating, to reminders of the traumatic event.

Avoidance symptoms:
- Making an effort to avoid thoughts, feelings, or conversations about the traumatic event.
- Making an effort to avoid places or people that remind you of the traumatic event.
- Having a difficult time remembering important parts of the traumatic event.
- A loss of interest in important, once positive, activities.
- Feeling distant from others.
- Experiencing difficulties having positive feelings, such as happiness or love.
- Feeling as though your life may be cut short.

Hypearousal symptoms:
- Having a difficult time falling or staying asleep.
- Feeling more irritable or having outbursts of anger.
- Having difficulty concentrating.
- Feeling constantly "on guard" or like danger is lurking around every corner.
- Being jumpy or easily startled.

You do not have to have all these symptoms to be diagnosed with PTSD. Diagnosis of PTSD typically requires a certain number of symptoms from each cluster. In fact, even if you don't have the minimum number of symptoms from each cluster, you can still be significantly suffering from symptoms related to your traumatic event(s).

Tool Application

There are numerous ways to educate and inform yourself about PTSD. Here are a number of ways to start this process:

1. The internet is full of information about PTSD. You can do a simple search by typing in PTSD and numerous pages with helpful information will appear. Of course, you will find some incorrect or poorly written information, but don't let this discourage you from continuing your search.

2. A lot of books, booklets and pamphlets have been written about PTSD. You can go to your local bookstore and browse what they have in stock or ask the clerk to do a computer search of books they can order. You can also directly order books yourself online from sites such as Amazon and Barnes & Nobles. Most of the books will let you examine the table of contents online as well as a selection of pages. Take time to find and order books that seem most helpful to you.

3. Attend local seminars on PTSD. Oftentimes local hospitals and mental health clinics will offer seminars on PTSD that provide good information. These seminars are designed as a community service and they are also designed to let you know about the services that hospital or clinic offers.

4. Attend a veteran's support group such as at a Vet Center that focuses on PTSD. Helpful information about PTSD is offered to newcomers who are learning about it.

5. Speak to your local chaplain or military mental health clinician about PTSD. They can provide knowledgeable information and material about PTSD. They can also help to diagnose whether you have PTSD and how severe.

Tool 2

Manage Flashbacks

A flashback is re-experiencing mentally the traumatic events that cause PTSD symptoms. Often the veteran feels and acts as if the traumatic event is happening again and may even lose awareness of the present moment. Not only is this emotionally and mentally overwhelming, but the person undergoing it often is anxious about the reaction of others around them who witness them experiencing a flashback, such as their spouse, children or friends.

Along with flashbacks, veterans may also experience dissociation, which is an experience in which they feel disconnected from themselves and their surroundings. With dissociation, like flashbacks, veterans may lose connection with events around them for periods of time in which they can recall nothing.

Flashbacks and dissociation are usually preceded by a *trigger*, or something that reminds them of the traumatic event and launches them into a flashback episode or dissociation. Triggers can affect any of the five senses including what the veteran sees, hears, smells, tastes or touches. For example, the smell of burning diesel can be a trigger. Witnessing a crime can be a trigger. Hearing a rifle go off while hunting can be a trigger. Attending a funeral in which taps is played can be a trigger. Many times triggers are unknown until experienced for the first time, and their effect can be overwhelming once a flashback or dissociation occurs.

Tool Application

There are several tools that you can use to limit or prevent the impact of triggers, flashbacks and dissociation:

1. Triggers are best managed by becoming aware of what your triggers are and then limiting your exposure to them or by learning to cope with them when they do occur. Often the only way you will know what your triggers are is by first experiencing them. Experiencing triggers the first time can be difficult, but is usually unavoidable as it happens unexpectedly, so when it does happen use that constructively as a learning experience. Once you know your triggers, you can seek to limit your exposure to those situations in which you know the trigger will be present. On the other hand, some individuals find when they absolutely can't avoid a trigger such as when they are at work, that repeated exposure to the trigger gradually increases their tolerance to it. Coping with triggers involves using all the other suggestions in this book such as talking with a trusted friend, using expressive writing and using relaxation techniques.

2. Identify early warning signs for flashbacks and dissociation. Sometimes it seems flashbacks and dissociation come out of nowhere, but closely examining what happens beforehand will often reveal warning signs. For example, you may start to feel fuzzy or dizzy or you may feel as though you are separating from your self. Around you everything may begin to take an unreal nature. You also may feel anxious and sense your heart beating faster. Identify as many typical warning signs as you can, and when you start to experience them use grounding, which is described next.

3. Grounding is a way of coping that keeps you in the present and helps prevent actively reliving a flashback or

dissociating. Just like one of your five senses experiencing a trigger, grounding uses the five senses to keep you solidly in the present.

- Sound: Turn on something loud. Loud music or talking is hard to ignore and helps to bring you back into the present moment. Be careful, however, if using ear buds not to damage your hearing.

- Touch: Hold on to something cold like an ice cube or cold drink. The coldness of the object will help you to stay in touch with the present moment.

- Smell: Sniff something with a strong smell such as vinegar. The strong smell helps to stay in the present like smelling salts help to bring around an unconscious person.

- Taste: Bite into something very tart or sweet. The tartness or sweetness of the sensation can force you to stay in the present moment.

- Sight: Start naming by name all the objects you see around you which will help keep you connected with the present.

Feel free to make substitutions to any of these so that they best fit your needs and situation.

4. Enlist the support of others to help you through your most challenging moments. Bring along a trusted friend at those times you think you might be most vulnerable to flashbacks or dissociation and tell them what to do to help you.

5. Seek professional treatment if the flashbacks and dissociation become debilitating and you need that extra support.

Ambushed!

The heat of the mid-August day and the smothering humidity had become almost unbearable for John. He stood chest high in brackish water as the marsh grass limped motionless in the still air. Since nine that morning, he had been working six hours straight and had only taken a brief break to wolf down some crackers and coke. Standing in the warm water on the Mississippi coast, he was struggling to nail some cross ties to the thick pressure treated posts that had been driven deep into the soft marsh mud. The temperature had reached nearly ninety-five degrees, but he still had several more cross ties to complete before he could call it a day. The stinging gnats and mosquitoes had not made his work any easier. His construction partner Vince had left an hour ago to go into town to buy some more construction supplies. They hoped to wrap up building the camp for their customer by the end of the week.

As he struggled for leverage to drive the thick long nail through the lumber, he suddenly caught movement out of the corner of his right eye. It appeared to be someone dressed in black disappearing behind a heavy growth of marsh grass. Though he was directly facing the shore, he turned his head in that direction to get a better look. At the same time, he caught more movement out of the corner of his left eye. Quickly turning his head in that direction, a wave of panic swept over him. Suddenly he heard the pop of an RPG being launched simultaneously with the intense crackle of small arms fire.

Instinctively, he threw himself under the muddy water as the thought raced through his mind "Ambush!" Fear gripped him as he realized he was all alone without his battle buddy and separated from his platoon.

Realizing he couldn't stay under water any longer, he burst through the surface and started flailing through the marsh grass to his right hoping to get out of the enemy's field of fire. The merciless onslaught of automatic weaponry and RPG fire continued in his direction and he was amazed he wasn't hit already. After ten minutes of difficult struggling through the thick marsh grass and mud, he managed to pull himself up onto solid ground near a grove of cypress trees. He took off running through the trees until he came to the one road in and out of the area. Yelling as he went to warn his fellow soldiers about the ambush, he thought it strange to see a red Ford truck coming down the road in his direction. Now feeling confused, he ran past the truck even as it slowed at his approach. He noticed that the driver was someone familiar, but not his battle buddy. In his mind the truck and the driver seemed somehow out of place, as if from a distant time.

The driver of the truck jumped out and started running back to him calling "John! John! What's the matter?" Recognizing the voice, John stopped and turned back to the man, frantically waving him back the other way, exclaiming they were being ambushed. The driver seemed confused by John's words. "Ambush? What do you mean? John, who's ambushing us? John are you okay?" Suddenly John knew something wasn't right. It finally hit him that the man was his construction partner Vince and this wasn't Vietnam. They couldn't be getting ambushed. John dropped to his knees with his hands to his face sobbing tears of disbelief at the experience he just had. Such an intense and realistic flashback had never happened to him before, though smaller less consequential flashbacks had occurred through the years. A couple of days later John made an appointment to talk with a counselor at the local Vet Center. He needed to deal with the past.

Tool 3

Monitor and Control Thoughts and Emotions

Learning to monitor and control your thoughts and emotions is crucial to controlling the symptoms of PTSD. First, though, you have to be convinced of the fact that you *can* control your thoughts and emotions rather than them controlling you. You may have felt up to this point that you cannot do anything to control the powerful thoughts and feelings you have been subjected to as a result of the traumatic experiences you previously encountered. But you can and you must. You *do* have the ability to be in charge of what your mind thinks and as a result what you feel. You cannot cause memories to disappear and past events to not have occurred, but you can control and change what you think about these and how you emotionally respond. You must believe this.

Second, as suggested above, it's important to understand that your emotions are closely tied to your thoughts. A thought that you have will usually have a related and accompanying emotion tied to it. For example, if you think on Saturday you will go and play a round of golf this will likely cause you to experience such emotions as happiness and excitement. Similarly, if you have the thought that tomorrow morning you are going out on military patrol in a dangerous part of the city, then you will likely have associated emotions such as anxiety, tension, fear and dread. Even more traumatic, let's say on your patrol an IED disables your vehicle, wounds members of your patrol, and the enemy pins you down with small arms fire. Though at the time you won't stop to evaluate your thoughts, they likely could include thinking that you may die, that your buddies may be killed, and that you won't see your family and loved ones again. Your training may prevent you from jumping up and fleeing, but emotions associated with your thoughts could possibly include terror, desperation, anger, despondency and fear of death and injury.

Weeks, months, and years later you may experience powerful thoughts and emotions related to your experiences that threaten to wreak havoc on your life. However, just like your training that prevented you from jumping up and running in the face of the enemy and increasing the chances of getting killed, so too can you train yourself to control your thoughts and emotions.

Tool Application

Without getting into too great of technical detail, outlined below is how to start the process of getting back in control of your thoughts and emotions.

1. First, you probably are more aware of your emotions and emotional reactions than you are your thoughts. You may be experiencing emotions and emotional reactions that are unwanted. As you learned above, however, your thoughts cause your emotions. You need to work backwards when you experience an unwanted emotion or emotional reaction and start asking your self "What thought or thoughts am I having that are causing the emotions I'm experiencing?" Usually these thoughts happen immediately before your emotional experience. You will have to rewind the "mental tape" in your head to identify these thoughts. For example, if you are back in the states and find yourself blocked in by traffic, you may begin to experience anxiety, nervousness,

and perhaps even panic. Your emotional reaction seems to you out of place compared to the situation. When you start to examine your thoughts then or later you realize that almost subconsciously you were thinking that being blocked in traffic is a potentially dangerous situation, because on your deployment it could make you a ripe target for an ambush or a vehicle borne IED.

2. After identifying the thought, now is the time to control it by challenging it mentally. You control the thought by challenging its truthfulness in your current life situation. Are you really in danger back in the states from an ambush or vehicle borne IED while stuck in traffic? The answer is no, unless perhaps you live in the most hardened and criminal parts of cities. You then need to replace it with a more accurate thought such as, "I don't like being stuck in traffic, but there is really no danger here." You will likely have to continue identifying and challenging thoughts over a longer period of time, and you may have to identify and challenge the same ones a number of times before you fully gain control over them. In effect, you are retraining your mind, and this takes time. As you challenge and overcome unwanted thoughts, you will find that your emotions begin to respond in a more favorable way and you have less and less unwanted emotions and emotional reactions.

Tool 4

Help Your Mind Help You

It is not uncommon to feel as if your mind is betraying you as you struggle to cope with PTSD. Your mind thinks in ways you often don't desire and you continue to have memories you would rather forget. It can be easy to conclude that your mind is on the verge of a break down. However, there is another way to look at the workings of your mind—a more constructive way. It can be helpful to compare your struggles to a laceration on your body. A small cut that only requires a Band-Aid is not going to create much pain and is not going to require much of your attention. Your body will heal the cut quickly. A large cut is a different story. You may require medical attention and you may be given stitches. You will have to care for it regularly. If you bump into something, it will cause a lot of pain and may start bleeding again. It will take the body much longer to heal. The important point though is that *the body is healing*.

Similarly, your mind heals as well, except that your mind's healing deals with your memories and emotions. A small mental injury, such as someone forgetting a dinner date with you will heal quickly and not create much difficulty. However, being in combat and witnessing or being a part of someone being killed or injured creates a memory that takes significantly longer to heal. Again, the important point though is that your mind is attempting to heal, though it often occurs slower due to the magnitude of the traumatic event. As your mind attempts to heal, it must return time and again to those traumatic events through memories and dreams in order to make sense of them, give them meaning, and to lay them to rest as much as possible. This can take a longer period of time the more traumatic the event. However, veterans sometimes lengthen this process by repressing their memories or covering them up though the use of alcohol or drugs. You need to help your mind help by actively contributing to the healing process and not avoiding it.

Tool Application

1. Accept that your mind has a way of healing as the body has a way of healing. Choose to help your mind in this process by proactively doing those things which will help it heal.

2. One way to proactively help your mind heal is to address your memories directly by writing about them, thinking about them, trying to understand what happened and why, and what meaning your experiences have for your life. If you feel directly addressing your memories is too threatening to do alone, then consider beginning this process with a counselor or friend helping. You may have to address the same memories numerous times before you begin to notice yourself coping better with them.

3. When experiencing unexpected disturbing thoughts or memories, remind yourself that they are part of the healing process. Your mind is at work even when you are not aware of it. When you unintentionally have these, then you may want to use their prompting to give thought to them and make sense of them at that time.

Convoy

The supply convoy was on its third and final day on the road heading from Kuwait to northern Iraq. The tanker trucks carried loads of diesel, a task which they had successfully accomplished many times before. SSG Gray sat in the passenger seat while PFC Jones took over the afternoon driving. The trip had been relatively uneventful. There were two long delays due to suspicions of IED's on the side of the road, but these proved to be simply roadside debris. The two soldiers were feeling a sense of relief that in approximately two hours they would be enjoying the comforts of the large base they were heading to.

As they passed by a cluster of trees growing close to the road, suddenly an RPG slammed into the cab of the truck on the driver's side. The explosion blew SSG Gray out of the cab and onto the ground below, but not before being peppered with shrapnel on his left side. Deaf from the explosion, he could see the truck slowly grinding to a halt in the shallow roadside ditch just ahead. Almost as soon as it stopped, he watched horrified as the cab of the truck burst into flames and slowly started to engulf it. Jerking himself to his feet, he shuffled as fast as he could up to the cab. He didn't hear the small arms fire going on about him, but another RPG round aimed at the disabled truck flashed overhead and he knew the convoy was still under attack. Grabbing hold of the truck, he pulled himself up on the cab step and peered in the open door. The intense heat was searing, and he could see that PFC Jones was slumped over the wheel fully immersed in the flames. He reached in desperately to grab hold of his arm to pull him out, but the fire burned him and the intense heat drove him back. Falling back off the truck cab on to the ground, he crawled away and took cover in the ditch. Sick with what he had just witnessed and weaponless, he remained motionless as the firefight raged about him. Twenty minutes later a military police patrol responding to the convoy's distress call rolled into view and helped drive the insurgents off.

Nine months later, Gray walked with his wife and son through the local community fair celebrating the Fourth of July. His return home had been a difficult one so far. He felt distant from his wife and had too frequently been short-tempered with his son. His wife had even suggested that he needed to seek help. At night he had been having nightmares related to his experiences and had taken to sleeping in another room so as not to disturb his wife. As night fell at the fair, the first volley of the firework display shot into the sky exploding in a beautiful display of reds, blues and whites. For Gray, however, the sounds and the sights were not so enjoyable. In fact, they were overwhelming and reminiscent of the sounds and sights in Iraq. Ducking instinctively to the ground and pulling his wife and child with him, he covered them with his body as surprised bystanders looked on nervously. His boy started to cry and his shocked wife trying to get out from under him kept asking what he was doing. The next round of fireworks intensified his feelings of danger, though his mind was telling him he was home from Iraq and was safe. It finally came to him that there was no danger, but due to the overwhelming intensity of the experience he remained lying on the ground sobbing with his face in his hands as his wife tried to help him. Someone ran and notified the paramedics who were on hand for the event, and they managed to guide him to the back of the ambulance until he was calmer. Returning home that evening, Gray agreed with the pleading of his wife that he needed help.

Tool 5

Address Guilt

Trauma survivors often find themselves struggling with trauma guilt. Veterans who experience trauma guilt have feelings of regret based upon the belief that there was something they should have or could have done differently at the time of the trauma. These feelings of guilt frequently leave the person feeling angry, upset, or ashamed of themselves. Feelings of sadness, depression, anxiety, low self-esteem, and even thoughts of suicide sometimes accompany guilt as well. Survivor guilt is a form of trauma guilt in which the veteran has made it through a particular traumatic event and others have not. The veteran questions and perhaps even blames him or herself about why they made it and others didn't.

Tool Application

1. Acknowledge your guilt. Guilt is something trauma survivors often feel but don't easily acknowledge. However, acknowledging your guilt helps to free your mind to cope with it. Acknowledging guilt involves two things: accepting that you are carrying around with you on a daily basis a sense of regret about the past and identifying those specific things you feel like you could have or should have done differently. Like other unpleasant thoughts, veterans often stuff deep inside any thoughts about guilt even

though the emotions are still tearing them up. By stuffing guilt, you are attempting to defend yourself against its tremendous mental and emotional impact on your life. But it is only by acknowledging the reality of your guilt and placing it directly before you that you are then ready to effectively deal with it. In acknowledging your sense of guilt, you may find it helpful to have someone else present to help you walk though it such as a chaplain, counselor, or friend.

2. Reflect on the true nature of the guilt. Traumatic events which affect your life are often so chaotic and so difficult to mentally grasp that sometimes you may blame yourself for things which can't reasonably be your fault or which you could not have realistically prevented. It is important to take time and thoroughly analyze your experiences, perhaps by writing the events down, and look at them as objectively as you can. It might be helpful to have another person help you in this process. Then ask questions such as, "What could I realistically have done or not done in that situation?" or "What would any other person have done in the same situation?" or "Are my thoughts and emotions any less different than others would have experienced?" By such an objective analysis, you may start to find that the guilt and blame you carry around is unwarranted.

3. Allow yourself to mourn. Guilt brings with it grief and sadness. Veterans grieve because of their losses. Mourning these losses is healthy and even essential for your healing. But not everyone mourns in the same way. Some cry, some withdraw, some talk to others, some grieve quietly. It is important though not to stifle your emotions, but to allow them to find expression in an open but safe way.

4. Choose to forgive yourself. The self-blame that comes with guilt is like beating yourself with a wooden club day

after day. Self-forgiveness reduces the harm of self-blame. Self-forgiveness starts with acknowledging the guilt and then becoming convinced of the truth that you are human and imperfect just like we are all human and imperfect. We all fail to live up to our expectations, and we fail more frequently in life-threatening situations. Self-forgiveness says that while I may continue to have thoughts and memories about the past, I forgive myself of my failures and imperfection and will no longer hold these against myself.

5. Choose to accept what cannot be changed. Part of moving forward in life is accepting that the past is the past and no matter how much you dwell on it there is not one single thing about the past that you can change. Dwelling on it, while understandable to a certain extent, drains your energy to make the most of the rest of your life. After having spent sufficient time to learn life lessons from the past and to make meaning of it as much as possible, it is then time to accept that the past cannot be changed. You may have to have little reminders to get yourself in a present and future pattern of thinking, such as post it notes or a message that pops up on your cell phone periodically.

Tool 6

Use Expressive Writing

Part of the struggle with PTSD is that veteran's memories, thoughts and feelings regarding their traumatic experiences often swirl in their mind at times as a bewildering mish-mash and at other times as sharp, extremely vivid and painful recollections. Sometimes the memories become intertwined and confused with other memories leaving veterans feeling uncertain about what really took place in their life and what didn't. Veterans also tend to interpret their memories and experiences in ways that emphasizes the worst leaving them feeling continually anxious, depressed and distraught.

Using expressive writing is a very good way to help cope with the impact of the traumatic event by taking control of your memories, thoughts, and feelings. When you write about your traumatic experiences, it helps you to think about the meaning of the trauma for your life, and it helps you to see it better for what it really is. As you write expressively, you may experience some uncomfortable emotions, but you will also notice that as you go along and complete each journal entry that the memories seem less and less threatening. In fact, expressive writing has been shown to help improve physical and psychological health.

Tool Application

1. Obtain a notebook or some loose leaf paper and find a quiet time and place where there are going to be few distractions.

2. Think about the traumatic experiences you have experienced and their impact on your life.

3. Begin writing in detail about those memories, thoughts and feelings you have from your traumatic experiences. Write about what happened to you. Write about their impact on your life. Write for at least 20-25 minutes.

4. Once finished, read over what you wrote and reflect on how your experiences now impact you emotionally and mentally. Think about the significance of your experiences for your life. Think about how your life is different, worse, and better as a result.

5. In doing this exercise you may experience some distressing thoughts and emotions. Be prepared ahead of time for how you might handle this distress, such as having a friend on hand or available to call and talk with.

6. Repeat this exercise for at least 2-3 more days. By doing this, you will find that your thinking becomes clearer and better organized and each time you get something helpful of the work.

Fallujah

Navy Corpsman Reed moved forward with the Marine platoon through the deserted and rubbled streets of Fallujah. Their company had been fighting for three straight days in the drive to retake the city from the insurgents. Already he had patched up and attempted to save more Marines than he cared to remember. The fighting had been fierce and relentless. They moved methodically from house to house sweeping their sector for the enemy. It was frustrating work. They would clear 20-30 houses, and then begin to relax thinking the insurgents had moved on to another sector, only to find a group of them strategically barricaded in another home. Even if the Marines took as many precautions as they could, someone still got killed or wounded.

As they moved up to a major street intersection everything seemed calm. The platoon paused to survey all the buildings and houses. Then a group of about nine Marines was sent scrambling across the street to the corner of a boarded up shop. Suddenly all hell broke loose. From atop the building across the street to the right and atop the building diagonally across the intersection insurgents opened up on the nine Marines and the rest of the platoon. Three of them went down immediately, while the others tried to shift for better cover. The rest of the platoon fired upward at the insurgents, but the enemy kept popping up and down keeping the Marines stifled. Then Corpsman Reed heard the words he had heard so many times, "Corpsman Up!" Reed zigzagged forward to the platoon leader who told him to cross the street and tend to the wounded Marines.

Not giving himself time to think about the danger, Reed stepped out from cover and started sprinting across the intersection. Only a few steps later, a bullet ripped through his knee. The shot dropped him stunned face down. Realizing he was not mortally wounded but still in the enemy's line of site, he struggled up on the good knee and drug himself the rest of the way across the street. Taking heavy bandages from his kit he managed to staunch the bleeding and pack the knee. He then started treating the fatally wounded soldier who had been pulled to cover and was even now talking his last breaths.

One year later, after a recovery at Bethesda Naval Center and a reconstructed knee, Corpsman Reed now served at a school to train other Navy corpsmen. While he was performing his duty well and the other corpsmen in training seemed to look up to him in awe, he was struggling. While he knew the procedures by heart, sometimes he would momentarily freeze up as flashes raced through his mind of treating all the wounded Marines on the battlefield. It was embarrassing when he had to be asked if everything was alright. He would snap back to reality and just blow it off as if he had been thinking.

He had also started drinking more and mixing his prescriptions. Several times he had fallen unconscious in his apartment. When he went out with his friends, which was rarely, he felt hyper guarded and was constantly in scan mode looking for dangers and threats where none could have reasonably existed. He constantly had a pervasive feeling that death could come at anytime, even though he was far away from the battlefield and would not be sent back due to his injury. He wondered if he could ever get back to the way he remembered himself before his combat experiences.

Tool 7

Build Resiliency

Resiliency is the personal capacity of people to positively cope with stress and traumatic events. Various personal factors affect how well a person copes with a traumatic event compared to another person. For example, a person who has experienced a previous traumatic event stands a good chance of coping better with another traumatic event than a person who has never experienced one before. The personal factors that affect how well we cope with stress and traumatic events are usually learned rather than inherited traits. It even appears possible that resiliency skills we learn after a traumatic event can be effective in helping us to cope with these past events.

Tool Application

Researchers have discovered a number of resiliency skills than can help veterans to better cope with present and past stress and traumatic events. Some of these are written about in more depth throughout this book, but there are also some other skills provided here. The more of these skills you learn, the better you will be at coping with past and future traumatic events.

1. The ability to cope with stress effectively and in a healthy manner. Think of your ability to cope with stress on a scale from constructive to destructive with various degrees

in between. Obviously, you will want to learn how to take stressful situations and make something constructive out of them. Too often though we allow stress to cause us to do destructive things to ourselves and those around us. Seek to learn better stress management skills such as relaxation skills and changing the way you think about situations.

2. Developing good problem-solving skills. Good problem-solving skills are helpful in countering the symptoms of PTSD. The more calmly and thoughtfully you approach problems in your life the more effective you will be able to resolve them. Learn to master problems though learning problem-solving skills rather than letting problems master you.

3. Holding the belief there is something you can do to manage your feelings and cope. There is a great difference between how a person responds to their PTSD thoughts and emotions who strongly believes he can improve them, and the person who does not. A positive, can-do attitude won't solve every problem, but it will help to solve more PTSD concerns than without it.

4. A willingness to seek help. Seeking help can be the hardest thing in the world to make yourself do. But once you have done it, you realize how good of a decision it was. Other people can offer much support and guidance if you will just be willing to let them. Perhaps the first person you seek help from won't be as helpful as you hoped, but don't let that be a discouragement. Keep seeking until you find the right person or organization, and then you'll realize the extra effort was worth it.

5. Being connected with others such as family or friends. PTSD often causes veterans to put up walls of isolation to others. This may be because they don't want others to see them struggling or how they have changed, but

being disconnected from others negatively affects their mental and emotional health. Start reestablishing these connections in order to promote your own recovery.

6. Self disclosure of your traumatic experiences to loved ones. One of the reasons veterans don't want to disclose their experiences to loved ones is that they believe no one will understand and they will reject you. While they may not fully understand everything, loved ones can still understand a lot. Like you, they are human too. They can also be compassionate, loving and supportive.

7. Spirituality. It doesn't take a study for a spiritual person to know the mental and emotional benefits of growing spiritually. However, a number of studies do concur with these benefits. Being spiritual is part of our nature, and if we encourage our own spiritual growth, the rest of us will grow and heal as well.

8. Having an identity as a survivor as opposed to a victim. Thinking of oneself as a victim leads to feelings of helplessness and forever being stuck in one's trauma. Thinking as a survivor leads to actively taking charge of your life and doing those things which will help in your recovery. Be a survivor, not a victim.

Avoidance

The Old Man

Hector had grown disillusioned with his deployment in Iraq. Decisions made and actions taken from the command level all the way down to his squad seemed senseless and counterproductive. Though he was only a PFC, he was bright and could see that their actions were only alienating the population from which they were supposed to be generating support. Back home in Puerto Rico, Hector had been studying music at the nearby university. Music had a harmony, a structure, a flow- but what they were doing here had none of that. On patrol, he saw his fellow soldiers treating the local Iraqis with disdain and contempt. Sometimes the soldiers would push, kick or hit the Iraqis if they didn't do what the soldiers indicated or if they didn't act quickly enough. By now most of the locals just went indoors when the American troops came by on patrol.

Two days ago, four soldiers in their sister company had been killed when they crowded around a man who spoke to them in broken English claiming to have information about anti-American fighters hiding nearby. When enough soldiers came close to the man, he blew himself up, killing the four and badly wounding six others. Now everybody was intensely on edge and mouthing threats of revenge on any Iraqi who came near them. The new orders were to shoot in self-defense any Iraqi who didn't halt when given the universal sign to stop. If the person kept coming, the soldier had the right to shoot.

As they set out that morning on their patrol, Hector didn't like the vibes he felt coming from some of the other soldiers.

Their threats and condemnations of the locals had reached such a fevered pitch he was certain something was not going to turn out right that day. As they moved into the center of the small town, Hector's squad leader told him to take up a position to the rear situated at a corner of an Iraqi home. The other soldiers moved forward to reconnoiter the area as he covered their rear. As he watched the soldiers move forward, he soon heard the shuffling of feet behind him. Walking towards him was an old Iraqi man holding up his hands and talking as if trying to ask Hector a question. At ten meters away, Hector raised his hand and told the man to stop in Arabic, one of the few words he knew. The man still kept coming, seemingly asking a question Hector couldn't understand.

Hector raised his weapon toward the man at the same time two members of his squad came walking up behind him. He yelled "Stop!" more forcefully hoping deep inside that the man would not continue coming forward causing him to have to fire. The man seemed to be slowing to stop, but one of the other soldiers yelled "Shoot him! Shoot him!" Hector held his fire, believing the man had understood him, but the soldier who was a sergeant continued to command him to shoot. Hector was now sweating and trembling, frozen with the decision. The old man suddenly lifted his hands and arms with his palms upward, as if cupping them. Hector fired. Three bullets tore through the man's chest and he dropped to the ground, wheezing for a few moments, and then died.

Four months later, after his redeployment, Hector lay motionless on his couch in his small apartment in Puerto Rico. Though unmoving on the outside, inside he was being ripped apart shred by shred by the guilt he carried with him everyday. At times he had thoughts of suicide, but he knew that was not the answer and went strongly against his religious beliefs. He had done little more than lay around his apartment since returning, and barely fed and cared for himself. Guilt was not an easy master.

Tool 8

Stop Avoiding

Avoidance of situations, memories or thoughts is a primary symptom of PTSD survivors. Veterans avoid certain situations, memories and thoughts because they are frightening and cause anxiety. The problems with avoidance are multifold. First, when veterans start avoiding things they begin to give up certain portions of their life, much of it formerly enjoyable. For example, they may avoid large groups of people because they feel uncomfortable or in danger, even if there is no true danger. As a result of this avoidance, they may no longer go to public events they used to enjoy, such as movies, sporting events, concerts and restaurants.

A second problem with giving in to avoidance is that it allows PTSD symptoms to hang around longer. When veterans avoid something they prevent themselves from overcoming that specific anxiety or fear by being exposed to it on a regular basis. For example, a veteran who experienced an vehicle borne IED attack on a crowded highway overseas may now avoid parts of their city or town that have high levels of traffic. They may find it difficult to travel to other places as well for concerns about crowded traffic there. However, if they convince themselves to increasingly commute in higher levels of traffic, they will find that their level of anxiety and fear begins to gradually diminish over time and they can drive just about anywhere they want. If they don't confront their avoidance though, their symptoms will last longer.

A third problem with avoidance is that one avoidance may lead to other avoidances and the quality of life become less and less. For example, a veteran may avoid going to funerals because it reminds her of the many memorials she attended while overseas. The avoidance of funerals may then generalize to avoidance of church because clergy are involved in funerals and churches often hold funeral services. Other related avoidances can also arise.

Tool Application

Avoidance related to PTSD is typically addressed with a trained therapist using exposure therapy. Exposure therapy is exactly as the name implies. In different ways it helps the person to safely confront those things which are causing anxiety and fear by exposing the veteran to them. By confronting those situations, memories and thoughts that cause anxiety and fear, the PTSD survivor will find that their symptoms begin to decrease on their own. It is recommended that exposure therapy be done with a trained therapist in order to properly train you on how it is done, guide you safely through the process, and make adjustments to ensure the most optimal outcome. Below are the three main forms of exposure therapy.

1. In Vivo exposure. In Vivo exposure involves the direct confrontation of the feared or anxiety provoking situation, activity, or object. Depending on the assessment by the therapist, In Vivo exposure can begin gradually and build up to directly confronting the feared activity, situation, or object or it can be done suddenly in a brief period of time. The therapist helps to ensure the confrontation is done safely and you have all the support you need.

2. Imaginal exposure. Imaginal exposure focuses on feared thoughts and memories. Sometimes it is not possible or not advisable to directly confront a feared situation,

activity, or object such as being in combat. Imagining oneself in the feared situation helps to better immunize the person to their fears by mentally exposing them to it.

3. Interoceptive exposure. Sometimes avoidance progresses to the point that veterans begin to fear experiencing their physical symptoms such as an increased heat rate or rapid breathing. Interoceptive exposure proceeds counter-intuitively by asking the person to purposefully attempt to exhibit the symptoms they are fearful of. For example, a person who fears their rapid breathing may be asked to breathe fast even when they are not having the symptoms. Often, the person finds their fear lessens and they are more in control of these symptoms.

4. Again, it is important to only attempt any of the exposure therapies in the presence of a trained therapist.

Tool 9

Renew Relationships

Social isolation is a common symptom of PTSD. Veterans experiencing PTSD often reduce contact with others. This is done to avoid situations that cause feelings of fear, embarrassment and anger, but isolation itself causes other major problems. It can result in the loss of social support, friendships and intimacy. It can also contribute to further depression and anxiety.

There are various levels and kinds of social isolation. Some social isolation may be as simple as not spending time with friends after work where in the past you would. It may involve remaining distant from family and not letting them get close to you to know what you are feeling and thinking. Social isolation can even go as far as withdrawing from society totally and avoiding any contact with other people. All of these, however, will have a harmful impact on your relationships and your mental and emotional health. Veterans all need some level of personal interaction and it only makes things worse when they avoid it.

Tool Application

The most effective way to overcome social isolation and its negative effects on your life is to make yourself become more active in interacting with others. Here are some different suggestions on how.

1. Renew your personal relationships with family and friends. Most veterans with PTSD still have some kind of relationship with someone, whether it is a son or daughter, wife or partner, an old friend or acquaintance. You must take the initiative to reconnect with these people and improve these relationships.

2. Increase contact with other veterans. Sometimes it feels like those who can best understand us are those who have been through something similar to what we have. There is a lot of truth in this. By joining a veteran's organization for vets and increasing contact with others who have experienced similar things to what you have, you can reverse the process of isolation. You will find that you feel better and have more satisfaction in life when you spend time with other veterans.

3. Join a PTSD support group. Joining a PTSD support group can be difficult because it means acknowledging publicly that you need help. This is understandable but should not prevent you from doing what will help get your life headed in the right direction. Remember, everyone else there had at one point or another similar thoughts and feelings to your own. As a result, they will be more understanding of your concerns. Once you start going, you will find it is very encouraging to know others who are struggling like you are and you can offer each other support and tips for how to better cope with PTSD. You may also develop life long friendships and relationships. By contacting your local VA hospital or Vet Center you will be able to locate PTSD support groups near you.

Predator

Lieutenant Colonel Manning stepped out of the air conditioned trailer into the Nevada desert heat and rubbed his eyes. It had been a long ten hour shift and a particularly disturbing one. The Predator Unmanned Aerial Vehicle he had been flying was now safely in the hands of the ground crew 7,000 miles away in Iraq. But he could not say as much for the supposed terrorist and bystanders he had just obliterated in a house in a remote Iraqi village. With a push of a button he had launched two Hellfire missiles on the structure and watched as it dissolved on the screen. The target in the house, he was told, was a high value al Qaeda operative who had eluded ground forces for nearly six months. When Lt. Col Manning guided the Predator over the target that intelligence had identified, he immediately noticed the women and children who were playing and working around the home. The vivid detail that the Predator's cameras provided left no doubt that *they were* women and children.

Manning relayed this information on to the decision makers and the decision had come back that the operative inside the house was of such high value that there might not be a chance to eliminate him again. He was ordered to take out the home, and if he could avoid the bystanders then do so. After the Hellfire missiles rained down and rendered complete destruction, Manning was certain innocents had been killed. Because he had to linger around in the air to asses the damage, the stark reality of how many innocents had been killed and wounded became clearly evident. Once his mission was complete, and the Predator landed, he tried to wipe the events from his mind. He needed too because he was now on his way back home to his wife and two little girls. This was becoming harder and harder as the number of missions continued to mount and were affecting his relationship with his family.

More and more at home, Manning withdrew to himself spending less and less time with his girls and his wife. When not sleeping, he would do the minimal required work around the house and watch long stretches of TV. It was as if he was there but not there. His girls learned that when pressed to spend time with them, he could become angry and snap, which was a definite change from his previous doting nature. His wife tried to point out how he was becoming increasingly distant and negative, but he replied that she should understand better the stresses of his work.

He had also started drinking greater quantities of beer during his off time, and there had been two or three occasions he had actually gone in to work still feeling the effects of the alcohol. Somehow he managed to hide it and had successfully completed his missions. Even at work he was becoming more distant from the other officers and NCO sensor operators. He talked less and seemed to be mechanical in his relations with others. Day-by-day the effects of his work as a Predator pilot were taking their toll, especially on his relationships, but Manning was struggling so much with his own conflicted emotions he didn't even noticed.

Tool 10

Be More Active

Post Traumatic Stress Disorder affects veteran's mood by causing them to feel more depressed or anxious. When your mood is affected in such a way you tend to be less likely to be involved in activities that you once enjoyed. If you are depressed as a result of PTSD, you often do not have the mental and emotional motivation to take part in normally enjoyable activities. If you are experiencing anxiety as a result of PTSD, you often avoid activities out of concern that they will provoke a flashback or that you will react in some unusual way that will cause us embarrassment in front of others.

Unfortunately, when veterans start to avoid activities that they once used to enjoy they eliminate those things from their life that may help to counter the depression or anxiety they are feeling. As a result, these feelings may only get worse. For example, a hungry person who avoids eating is only going to feel hungrier. A depressed person who avoids pleasurable activities is only going to feel more depressed. A person with anxiety who avoids activities and people because of their anxiety will feel more anxious the next time they are encountered.

Tool Application

1. The key here is to make yourself get involved in life's activities. You won't feel like being more active, but don't

give into this feeling. Sometimes a car that is stalled only needs to get rolling first before the clutch can be popped to get it started. The more ways you are active in your life that are pleasurable or enjoyable the more your mood will improve.

2. It is important to have a variety of activities. If you try just one thing and it doesn't seem to help, you may then think that nothing will help. Even if that one activity does seem to help, the improvement may be limited. It is better to choose activities from several different areas such as hobbies, sports, career, spirituality, education, relationships, health, travel and others that might personally interest you.

3. Instead of just picking activities and jumping in, you may find it even more helpful to set some goals. For example, if you choose education, a goal might be to complete a bachelors or masters degree. If you choose health, a goal may be to lose a certain amount of weight. If you choose spirituality, a goal may be to join a bible study group. Goals are important because they help to increase your commitment to whatever activity you choose.

4. Once you have chosen your goals, you will likely find it beneficial to track your progress. Tracking your progress simply means identifying what you have done each week toward achieving your goal. You can do this mentally or you can keep track of it on a calendar or a daily tracker. You will find satisfaction and be able to measure your progress by looking back over your activities and seeing how far you have come.

5. You should start off any new activities slowly and with reasonable goals in mind. If you set goals that are too ambitious and cannot achieve these, you will experience an emotional and mental setback. Start out with some goals and activities that have some challenge to them

but are achievable. For example, if you are seeking to complete an educational degree you might want to start out with taking just a couple of classes the first semester, then building up to a fuller load.

6. If you run into any problems achieving the goals you set, take a look back and see if there were any obstacles or unexpected events that prevented this. Problem-solve the best way to resolve or avoid these problems should they arise again. Being more active in your daily life is a great way to improve your mood and find direction for your life.

Tool 11

Emphasize the Positive

Traumatic combat experiences seem to leave little room in veteran's lives for anything except the struggle with the aftermath. However, researchers are beginning to discover that many veterans can emerge from traumatic experiences with greater self-confidence, a keener sense of compassion, and appreciation of life. These personal growth outcomes are in no way meant to downplay the negative impact of PTSD, but they do offer a more hopeful way to cope.

Sometimes when veterans are faced with the heavy burdens of life and their traumatic experiences, they neglect to notice that they have grown and matured as a person. As a result, they miss out on an important avenue for recovery. For example, let's say two service members were involved in the exact same traumatic combat event. One interprets the situation more with a focus on how it has helped him improve his leadership skills and how he now appreciates life more. The other focuses more intently on the near traumatic ending of his life and the senselessness of it all. Which seems more likely to have a better mental and emotional outcome? The first of course. This is not to say the first won't also have PTSD symptoms later on, but there is a good chance they will be less severe and debilitating.

The point is that it is up to the individual veteran to give significance and meaning to the events in their life. The significance and meaning that you give to traumatic combat experiences will likely impact how well or how poorly you cope with these experiences.

Tool Application

Here are a couple of simple exercises that you can do to help yourself begin to discover what is meaningful and positive in your traumatic experiences.

1. Write down ways that you feel you are different now as a person as a result of going through your traumatic experiences. List as many positive ways you are different as you can think of. Focusing on each of the positive ways you are different; write down for each how these are evident in your life. For example, if a positive is that you are more compassionate toward others, write down specific ways that you find yourself being more compassionate toward others. Then write down other ways you could potentially be more compassionate toward others. Finally, select some of the new potential ways to be compassionate and make a commitment to do more of these in your daily life.

2. Similar to the exercise above make a list of ways you are different in an undesired way as a result of your traumatic experiences. Examine each closely and ask yourself how each one may possibly be turned into something positive. Not all of those that you list will you be able to turn it into something positive, but for many you will. For example, let's say one of the things you list is that you are isolating yourself from others. This is generally not desirable as regular interpersonal contact is important for good mental and emotional health. However, you can turn this into something positive by using your time alone to read books about improving yourself and your relationships. Not only will you learn new personal and relational skills, but you will also likely become more motivated to engage in relationships to practice these skills.

Chopper Down!

Word came over the Singars radio to Bravo Company of the heavy engineering battalion that a CH-47 Chinook had gone down in their sector and they were to respond immediately to help secure and recover the wreckage. The company was located in a forward location in Afghanistan to prepare a base from scratch for a follow on brigade size element of infantry. It was part of the new push into the more remote regions to root out the insurgents. Bravo Company had only been at the new site for two weeks when the word came about the Chinook. First Sergeant North was to lead a fifty man outfit to the wreckage to secure it and search for survivors until a larger body could arrive. The company commander would stay behind with the rest of the company.

The drive over the rough terrain to the site took half an hour and gave 1SG North time to prepare for what they might encounter. Once they arrived, however, it was worse than he thought. The helicopter had hit hard and much of it was pulverized into small pieces and was still smoldering. After establishing the perimeter, 1SG North and ten other soldiers started combing the crash. There appeared to be no survivors, but the physical condition of the dead was overwhelming. The occupants of the helicopter had been rendered and torn apart by the impact with the ground. Their remains lay scattered about among the charred metal pieces of the Chinook. The smell of death was noxious and unforgettable. Particularly disturbing scenes of death from the sight etched themselves in North's mind, and he knew they would stay with him for a very long time. Finally, after a grim but thorough search, North pulled the searchers out of the carnage and sent them to help man the perimeter until further help arrived.

Nine months later as they were redeploying, 1SG North sat in a small office with a representative from the VA sitting across from him. "First Sergeant, on the questionnaire you filled out for us as part of the redeployment process, it shows that you're experiencing some symptoms of PTSD," the VA representative was saying. "It suggests you're having difficulty with memories of your experiences, anxiety, and trouble sleeping." North couldn't be more irritated and annoyed. He felt his anger rising. The last thing he needed was to get delayed at this stage of returning home, and not get to see his wife and children in two days. "Your questionnaire must be wrong," North said flatly. He knew it was probably right as he had answered as truthfully as possible, but he didn't expect to get held up now. He thought that later if his symptoms continued to get worse, his responses would support his need to receive treatment. But now this man was the only thing standing in the way between he and his family. "Actually the questionnaire has been tested over many years and found highly reliable, as long as you answered honestly," the VA representative assured him. North felt cornered now. He knew he probably needed treatment, but he didn't want it now. He didn't want to be sent off to some medical center at another fort to await treatment for months on end. The representative sensed his anxiety and guessed his concerns. "Look. I know you just want to go be with your family now. I don't want to prevent that. What I'm trying to do is identify those who need the help. We can arrange for you to see someone later, once you come back from your leave. And we don't have to send you off anywhere. We have counselors here on post who can talk with you on an outpatient basis and it's all confidential. In the meantime, we can ask the chaplain to come by and follow up with you to

make sure everything is going okay. How does that sound?"
North liked that plan much better. Already he felt some relief
that he would be able to talk with someone about the mental
and emotional struggles he was having with the experiences
from his deployment. Now he could focus on enjoying his
reunion with his loved ones.

Tool 12

Acceptance

People naturally tend to avoid things that cause pain. Pain however is a part of life and it is not completely avoidable no matter who you are or what you do. Some people are in positions and professions in life in which they will be more likely to encounter experiences that cause pain than other people are. Military service members are one such group of people. The more traumatic the experience people have the more intense the emotional and mental pain usually is. Even after the experience has passed, individuals still have reminders of the experience whether it is events, smells, sounds, sights or memories. These reminders often bring up the pain afresh and anew. In order to prevent this, individuals often do whatever they can to avoid these reminders and thus avoid the pain.

While the avoidance of pain is natural and understandable, it is not effective at alleviating suffering. Veterans try to avoid their pain in different ways, many of which are counter-productive, such as drinking, drugs, self-harm, and relational conflicts, among others. Avoiding the pain of PTSD is like having a large cut on your arm and running as fast as you can hoping to get away from the hurt. The pain stays with you no matter how fast you run. Accepting your experiences and pain is a more effective way for reducing the impact of them on your life. The process, however, does not stop with acceptance. It also includes committing yourself to identifying and achieving the values that you find important in life.

Tool Application

1. Take an accounting (preferably on paper) of those past experiences you have been actively avoiding being reminded of and re-experiencing. Also, take an accounting of the pain that the reminder of these experiences causes for you. How do they make you feel? What thoughts do they make you have, including about yourself? Be honest with yourself about what the experiences are and the pain they cause that you have been avoiding.

2. Accept that these experiences truly happened and there is no way to change this fact. Accept that it is normal for you, and for anyone, to experience the emotional and mental pain you have. Accept that no one is perfect and anything you did or didn't do could have easily been repeated by anyone else. Accept that avoiding the experience and the pain only causes the healing to be delayed that much longer. Accept anything else that you know you have been trying to avoid that is real and true about your experiences.

3. While accepting the truth of your experiences and pain, challenge those thoughts about your experiences that are not reasonably true. For example, if you have thoughts about being guilty for something regarding your experiences, question the thought and determine whether it is a true guilt or false guilt (see Tool 5 on guilt).

4. End the struggle based on the avoidance of your experiences and pain. Do not continue to war within yourself. Accept your experiences and pain for what they are.

5. Commit yourself to using the energy that you once used in avoiding your experiences and pain to identifying and achieving those values that you find important in life.

6. Identify what things are important to you and establish a present and future focus on achieving those things that you value. Accept that some greater or lesser degree of pain concerning the past will always be part of your life, but commit to spending more energy and focus on the present and future than on the past.

Tool 13

Develop a Daily Activity Plan

The debilitating effects of PTSD often make it difficult to establish goals, create a daily routine, and be productive in life. Sometimes PTSD makes veterans feel as if they are caught in quicksand causing their every move to seem as if it is in slow motion and sapping their energy. Sometimes veterans struggle just to force themselves to get up in the morning from a restless night and seem able only to take care of their most basic needs, and possibly to muddle through work that day.

Part of the problem in being unfocused and unproductive is that you need more structure to get yourself going and keep yourself going. PTSD is notorious for keeping veterans bogged down in the mire and muck of their experiences. What is needed is to develop daily activity plans that will help you get up and moving and achieve your short-term and long-term goals.

Tool Application

The following are steps to take to help you establish goals, create a daily routine and be more productive in your life.

1. Start with identifying what is important for you and your life. Ask yourself questions such as these to help with this: How would you evaluate you life right now? How is your job? Are you content? Are you where you

want to be? Do you want to be more involved in your community? Does that mean joining a church, a social group, or volunteering somewhere? Do you want to take up any new hobbies or start a craft? Do you want to go back to school? What do you want to study? Do you want to improve your relationships? Have you wanted to start working out? Does that mean joining a gym or a weight-loss program? Think of other questions that best addresses who you are and what you want to do in life. Rank items by what is the most important to you.

2. Take the answers to the above questions and restate them as goals. For example, if you want to change career paths by obtaining a college degree, you might state it as: "My goal is to complete a business degree in four years. I will do this my using my GI Bill benefits and continue to work part time in my present job." Restate your answers as goals for each one ranked in order of most importance to least importance. Make sure your goals are realistic, achievable, and do not conflict with your other goals.

3. Now looking at each goal, determine what must be done each month, each week and each day in order to achieve them. This will also be helpful in being able to seek whether you have too many or too few goals by how much you can reasonably accomplish in a month, week, and day. Your daily activity plan should have a number of actions you should be taking each day to work toward your goals. The daily activities should be scheduled out on something like a daily planner so you know at what times you need to be where doing whatever the activity you planned for that time. You should be flexible with the planning of your daily activities to make necessary changes while still remaining focused on achieving your goals.

4. Take time to review after each day, each week, each month, and each year to determine whether you are successfully on track toward achieving those goals you set. Make appropriate adjustments as needed.

Hyperarousal

Alone

Specialist Morgan stepped out the back of the movie theatre on the former Iraqi post. It was already past 1200 and the air was still hot in the June night. She carried two large black bags of trash she had collected and was taking them to the dumpster out back. Normally, she would be in her bunk fast asleep at this hour, but her First Sergeant had informed her she was chosen to pull special duty at the post theatre that night. The door closed behind her and the only sound she could hear was the loud reverberating of the large generator behind some HESCO barriers that powered the theatre. A weak light illuminated the back of the building and she could see just enough to locate the dumpster the NCO in charge of the theatre had told her would be there.

A large crowd had been present for the two showings of the movie that night, and some of them had acted rowdy. But that was understandable as this was one of the few places where they could relax and be themselves. Every thirty minutes she was required to make rounds in the theatre with a flashlight as the movie was showing in order to make sure everything was in order. While it wasn't uncommon for guys to flirt with her, she sensed one guy staring intently at her in a way that made her feel uncomfortable.

After pitching the bags in the dumpster, she turned to go back inside but suddenly heard the quick movement of feet behind her and then the powerful grip of an arm around her neck and hand across her mouth. Even worse she felt the sharp point of a large knife against her ribs.

"If you scream I'll kill you! You understand?" the husky voice threatened with utmost believability. Though in shock, Morgan nodded knowing the attacker was serious. Even if she could scream, the noise of the generator would have muffled any sound. "Do everything I say and you'll get out of this alive. Don't ever look at me. Got it?" Specialist Morgan could only nod again.

Remaining behind her the attacker ordered her to strip her pants down to her boots and get on the ground. He then proceeded to rape her. She could only sob silently during the attack fearful that she would still be killed. After the rape, the attacker left quickly telling her to keep her face on the ground until he was gone. Minutes passed and she finally found the courage to get up and flee. Leaving the theatre, she ran back to her bunk and awoke her best friend and battle buddy trying to tell them what happened through her intense sobbing. Her friend convinced her to go to medical where she was checked out and a rape kit done. A couple of days later she agreed to meet with a counselor. The counselor, however, seemed to be overwhelmed with other soldiers and not as understanding as Morgan thought she would be. She didn't go back.

Specialist Morgan heard little about the investigation into who the perpetrator was except that they hadn't found the guy. She found herself struggling with falling asleep, depressed feelings, crying spells and trouble concentrating. She was making mistakes in her responsibilities as a personnel clerk, though the senior NCO was understanding. She especially struggled with concerns about safety, and would not go anywhere around the post without her battle buddy. Much of the time that she was not working she stayed closed up in her bunk. Whenever she had to go out, such as to the chow hall, her friends noticed that she was extremely jumpy and on guard. Her symptoms had become so severe she didn't know how she could complete the remaining seven months on her tour. Time had become unbearable.

Tool 14

See Things for How They Really Are

All of your experiences in life shape how you see and interpret events on a daily basis. For example, if you were once mugged while taking a walk in a seemingly safe city park, you may naturally begin to think of parks as dangerous places. In the same way, if you experienced life-threatening encounters while deployed, then you may begin to think and feel that certain similar situations back home are life threatening or at least a threat. It is as if you have put on a pair of glasses with your past experiences etched on them. As you try to go about your daily life once back home, you continue to see much of your everyday experiences through these lenses. However, what you see is sometimes not the way things really are.

The effect of not seeing things as they really are is that you think, feel, and react in ways that are not equivalent to what the reality of the situation is. You may respond in a way similar to how you responded in the past to a life threatening or traumatic event. Your response may be overly defensive, angry, self-protective, violent or helpless. Since your responses may be disproportionate to the current situation, they can lead to troubled relationships, social embarrassment, and legal scrapes among others. Obviously you will want to adjust the way you are seeing things, if this is happening.

Tool Application

1. Identify what situations currently cause you to experience thoughts, feelings and actions that seem over reactive and out of place. In these situations you may perceive some danger to yourself or others.

2. On a piece of paper draw five columns. In the first column put a heading of "Situation." In the second column put a heading of "Thoughts." In the third column put a heading of "Response." In the fourth heading put a heading of "New Thoughts." In the fifth column put a heading of "New Response."

3. Under the "Situation" heading write down in a few words what the situation was that caused you to react the way you did. Next to that under the "Thoughts" heading write down what thoughts you remember having immediately after you encountered the situation. Next to that in the "Response" column write down what response to the situation you had that was undesired. Next, in the "New Thoughts" column write down what would have been more fitting thoughts that would have better matched the reality of the situation. Finally, in the "New Response" column write down what would be a more fitting and constructive response or responses to the situation based upon the new thoughts you identified. Review your work until you feel confident about your responses.

4. Do this exercise for each new situation you encounter in which you do not feel that your thoughts, feelings and responses match the reality of the situation. Save your work and continue to review it over time to help the new thoughts and new responses become a part of your everyday life.

Tool 15

Train Yourself to Relax

PTSD often causes veterans to go about their day with an ever present feeling of anxiety and tension. Due to this heightened arousal veterans tend to overreact to events in their daily life potentially causing problems in their relationships and work. Training yourself to relax on cue is an excellent way to lower your anxiety and tension as well as your arousal level. Described below you will find outlined a tool called Progressive Muscle Relaxation. Progressive Muscle Relaxation teaches veterans how to control their anxiety and tension levels by relaxing their body and mind. It requires about 30-45 minutes at first to complete the exercise, but each time you do it you get better skilled and your body responds more quickly. Eventually you can even be in a group of people and still be able to relax your body and mind using a shortened version of this tool.

Tool Application

1. Start by getting into a comfortable position. A comfortable chair is ideal. Close your eyes. Place your feet flat on the floor, legs uncrossed and your hands resting comfortably at your side or on your lap.

2. Begin by noticing your breathing, noticing your abdomen rise and fall with each breath (pause after each breath). As your breathing becomes more relaxed and restful, take

your awareness up to your face. Then you'll start this process with the muscles in your face.

3. Tense the muscles in the face by making a sour face, like you just ate a lemon, holding that face for four seconds and then release the muscles in your face. Repeat the process two times in various muscle groups throughout the body.

4. Notice the tension just washing away. With each tense and release cycle, you'll notice it becomes easier and easier to release and relax each muscle group. Do the same thing you just did before, except you should be inhaling through the nose and exhaling through the mouth, relaxing even more with each breath.

5. Now, you should move your awareness to the shoulder and neck area. Notice the muscles in the shoulder and neck area. Tense the muscles in the neck by pressing the shoulders towards the ears and holding for a count of four seconds and then release. With your awareness in the neck and shoulders, now tense them and hold for four seconds, and release. Notice the difference between a tense muscle and a relaxed muscle as you go through the process. Remember to inhale through the nose and exhale through the mouth, releasing any residual tension in this area. Do it again, relaxing even more with each breath.

6. Bring your awareness to the muscles in the arms. Tense the muscles in both of your arms by curling the arms up towards your biceps and holding them as if you are lifting weights and holding them to your chest, holding for four seconds and then release. With your awareness in the arm, do the same thing again. Remember to inhale through the nose and exhale through the mouth, can release any residual tension in the arm. Do it again, relaxing even more with each breath.

7. Now, bring your awareness to the muscles in the hands. Tense the muscles in the hands by clenching it into a tight fist, holding for a count of four seconds and then release. With your awareness in the hands, now tense the muscles in your hands and hold for four seconds and release. Notice the tension just wash away when you release. Do it again, relaxing even more with each breath.

8. Notice the muscles in the upper back, around the shoulder blades. Tense the muscles in the upper back by pressing the shoulder blades together and holding for a count of four seconds and then release. With your awareness in the shoulder blades, now tense and hold for four seconds, and release. Notice the difference between tensed muscles and relaxed muscles as you go through the process. Do it again, relaxing even more with each breath.

9. Now, notice the muscles in the abdomen and low back. Tense the muscles in the abdomen by imagining that you are trying to touch the belly button to the spine, pressing the lower back to the chair and holding for a count of four seconds and then release. With your awareness in the abdomen, now tense and hold for four seconds, and release. Notice the difference between a tense muscle and a relaxed muscle again. Remember to inhale through the nose and exhale through the mouth, releasing any residual tension in the lower back and abdomen. Do it again, relaxing even more with each breath.

10. Now on to the feet. Tense these muscles by pointing the toes towards the knees, and again holding for three seconds, and then releasing the calf muscles. With your awareness in the calf muscles, now tense the calves and hold for four seconds, and release. Notice the difference between a tense muscle and a relaxed muscle as you go through the process. Remember to inhale through the

nose and exhale through the mouth releasing any residual tension in the calves. Do the same thing you did before again, relaxing even more with each breath

11. Eventually, after you practice this procedure enough, you will be able to bring yourself to a deep state of relaxation by simply telling your whole body to relax at once like you do step-by-step as you go through the process. Be sure you do this procedure only in a safe place and not while you are driving or operating machinery. It is helpful to do this exercise by having someone slowly read it out loud while you respond.

Tool 16

Practice Mindfulness

Mindfulness is a tool that emphasizes being completely in touch with the present moment. Veterans with PTSD often find that their thoughts, particularly the disturbing ones, seem to take control over their lives and create everyday living problems for them. Mindfulness helps you to take a step back from your thoughts and reduces their power to negatively impact your life. You may desire to have a friend or therapist present to help guide you safely through the process when you first attempt it.

Tool Application

1. Find a comfortable position either lying on your back or sitting. Close your eyes and relax your muscles allowing all tension to leave your body.

2. Spend time focusing on your breathing. Focus on the rise and fall of your chest and imagine you are riding on a wave of air you breathe in and out.

3. Now turn your attention to the thoughts that are entering your mind. You can imagine your thoughts as an object gently floating through you mind such as a leaf floating on the breeze or a snowflake gently floating by. Do not try to control your thoughts or linger on them. Just allow them to pass through as you observe them going by.

4. You may notice yourself from time to time getting immersed in your thoughts. This is normal. Try to determine what it is about the thought that caused you to become immersed in it and then return back to simply observing your thoughts.

5. After a few minutes of observing your thoughts, return your focus back to your breathing and open your eyes when you are ready.

6. Practice this tool everyday and you should begin to notice you are more in control and at peace with your thoughts.

Beginners Mind

Beginners mind is a variation of mindfulness that emphasizes looking at thoughts as if you are seeing them for the first time. It can help to enhance the mindfulness tool by allowing more evaluation of the thoughts that pass through your mind. After practicing and becoming skilled at mindfulness, incorporate the following two extra steps:

7. As your thoughts pass through your mind start to examine them more closely. Notice exactly what the thought is. Notice how each particular thought has an impact on your life. You can choose to speed up or slow down the thoughts as they pass.

8. Continue to really examine the thought. Do you notice anything about it and its meaning for your life that you had not noticed before? How does the thought relate to your combat experiences and symptoms of PTSD? Does it contribute to the symptoms or help prevent the symptoms? Does the thought need to be challenged and corrected.

The Sandman

Sleep had become the best friend as well as the worst enemy for Josh. For seven months since his return from Afghanistan as a Marine combat veteran, he had gotten at most only a few good nights of sleep. While he desperately wanted and needed to sleep, his constant dreams and the associated anxiety left him fitfully tossing and turning at night.

His surreal dreams frequently took him back to the small outpost in a remote Afghanistan mountain village he and a small number of other Marines manned most of his time there. Attacks were a near daily occurrence and a number of his friends were airlifted out in body bags or stretchers during his tour. One day as he was returning to the outpost from patrol, his squad was suddenly and violently attacked on three sides by Taliban insurgents. Above him on the rocky slope an RPG was fired. The rocket sizzled toward him at unimaginable speed and ricocheted off his Kevlar helmet shattering it to pieces. An insurgent then burst out running from behind a stone outcropping and rushed up to him directly pointing his AK-47 at Josh's chest. He fired twice. The armor plating in his body armor cracked but stopped the bullets, leaving him with only a badly bruised sternum. A fellow Marine shot the insurgent before he could fire again. The squad managed to fight off the insurgents with the help of air cover and another detachment from the outpost. Josh was eventually sent to the rear and on to Germany to be further evaluated for brain damage, due to symptoms he started experiencing.

After an honorable discharge, Josh and his wife and son moved back to their hometown in the Midwest. Receiving treatment from the VA, Josh was unable to work due to his lingering brain damage. Short-term memory loss made it impossible to find work that he could reliably perform. Not long after he returned home, his sleep problems began. He started having vivid dreams. One such dream involved running through an Afghanistan village with his wife and child trying to protect them while insurgents fired at them from all sides. He would wake up sweating and trembling and could not sleep any further that night. Even though he was taking six pills a day to help sleep, their effectiveness was minimal and his wife felt he was becoming dependent on them.

Anxiety about going to sleep also became a problem. While he wanted to sleep, anxiety about the dreams created conflict within him of wanting sleep but avoiding it. Frequently, he would stay up to 2 a.m. watching television before he would go to bed hoping that this somehow would cause himself to be less likely to dream. It didn't help, but did reduce his sleep even more. The lack of sleep made him more irritable during the day, and made his already impaired ability to think even worse. He seemed to be caught in a vicious cycle in which the very thing he needed the most seemed harder and harder to get.

Tool 17

Prepare to Sleep Better

Veterans sometimes have sleep problems related to their traumatic experiences. Trouble sleeping is one of the most common problems PTSD survivors experience. Sleep problems can include trouble either falling asleep, staying asleep, or both. Sleep problems generally occur due to feelings of hyper-arousal. Feeling hyper-aroused is a result of the thoughts and emotions veterans continue to have related to their PTSD. A lack of sleep leads to further problems such as stress, mood problems, as well as negatively affecting your health. It is important to start taking some positive actions which will help you better prepare for a good night's sleep.

Tool Application

Here are some things you can do to help improve your sleep.

1. Exercise during the day. However, make sure to avoid exercise within six hours of your bedtime.

2. Try to stick to a regular sleep schedule. Make it a habit to get up at the same time in the morning and try to go to bed around the same time each night.

3. Reduce the amount of caffeine and nicotine that you consume during the day. Avoid drinking caffeine after lunch time, and do not smoke before going to bed.

4. Try to avoid or limit naps during the day, especially after 2 p.m.

5. Avoid consuming alcohol within six hours of your bedtime.

6. Forcing yourself to fall asleep will never work. If you are having a hard time falling asleep after 20 to 30 minutes, get up out of bed and try to do something relaxing. Reading a book is an excellent way to gently tire the mind for sleep, as long as the book is not too exciting and intense. Avoid watching television. Do not return to bed until you feel drowsy.

7. Try to make your bedroom a relaxing place, and try to limit your activities in the bedroom. For example, do not eat, watch television, check e-mail on your laptop, or talk on the phone in bed. Your bedroom should be associated with sleep.

8. Try to keep your bedroom at a cool and comfortable temperature.

9. Utilize a white noise machine, ear plugs, or an eye mask to help block out any distracting noises or light.

10. Practice relaxation exercises before bed to release muscle tension and slow down your breathing.

11. Lower the lighting an hour or so before going to bed. This helps to cue your body that you are ready for sleep.

12. Use medications for sleep cautiously and only under a physician's supervision.

13. Find ways to express and process unpleasant emotions and thoughts before going to bed. Some sleep problems may be due to not adequately coping with stress. Journaling

can be a helpful way to express and process these emotions and thoughts in a positive manner.

14. If intrusive thoughts and memories related to your traumatic experiences are preventing you from falling asleep or waking you up, then spend time during the day and before you go to bed practicing some of the tools in this book dealing with monitoring and controlling your thoughts, relaxation, and helping your mind help you.

Tool 18

Take a Break from Anger

Anger is an emotion that serves a constructive purpose when used appropriately and in the right circumstances. Anger serves to prevent further hurt or harm to come to yourself or others. Veterans with PTSD symptoms, however, may find that their anger seems to be ever present and a destructive force in their life. It can lead to unnecessary conflicts and arguments with others as well as professional problems such as problems on the job. In severe cases, anger can even escalate into violent behavior. As a result, it is important that you learn to take a break from your anger in order to avoid having it get out of control.

Various ways exist to manage anger. For example, the use of relaxation techniques such as deep breathing and relaxing imagery can help to calm down angry feelings. Changing the way you think is another by altering those thoughts that lead to anger such as "He is trying to embarrass me" or "Why can't she do anything right?" Another way is through problem solving which seeks to calm anger by solving the problems that frustrate you.

Taking a break or a timeout from anger is another way to control your emotions and helps to put you in a better state of mind. It can be done immediately when you start to notice yourself becoming angry.

Tool Application

1. Taking a break or a timeout from anger means temporarily removing yourself from an escalating situation so you can cool down.

2. Develop a plan beforehand of what you are going to do and where you are going to go should you need to take a break. Typically, you should identify a place that is quiet and relaxing for you. You should also have some skills to help you calm down during that time such as breathing deeply or closing your eyes and thinking about a relaxing place such as a tropical island with waterfalls.

3. Train yourself to recognize the signs that you are getting angry. For example, you may start to feel warm and your heart may beat faster or you may feel your muscles tightening.

4. When you notice your anger is increasing, remove yourself from the situation as soon as you are able. Leave the situation well before your anger boils over. If you are talking with another person you may simply need to excuse yourself.

5. After you are away from the situation and in a quiet place, focus on your relaxation techniques such as deep breathing or relaxing imagery. Make sure you don't spend the time negatively ruminating about the situation.

6. When you feel you have successfully calmed yourself down, think about the situation and how you can handle it more positively. Then return to the situation and handle it in that more positive way.

7. Keep in mind that taking a break should only be temporary, and if sufficiently calm you should return to the situation and attempt to resolve it.

8. Continue to learn other ways to manage anger as the more skills you have the better.

9. Consider practicing this tool before hand so you'll be prepared when the situation arises.

Tool 19

Increase Positive Distracting Activities

Sometimes when struggling with the memories, thoughts and feelings associated with PTSD, veterans temporarily need something that will distract them and give them a moment of rest. The intensity of the thoughts and feelings within the veteran can be overwhelming, and the veteran needs something to help settle him or herself down, even if only for a short period of time. This break from these PTSD symptoms can help you regain the mental and emotional energy needed to continue to directly cope with your symptoms. Positive distraction alone is unlikely to facilitate recovery but it can serve as a "breather" to help you regain your inner composure and move forward with your life.

Positive distraction works by taking your mind off of a strong emotion or thought and by focusing it on something else that interests you. Sometimes when you focus on a strong emotion or feeling it can seem much worse. Positive distraction is different from negative distraction in the sense that positive distraction benefits you and negative distraction typically harms you. For example, drugs and alcohol are negative distractions that ultimately harm veterans and prevent them from moving forward with healing. Positive distraction, on the other hand, facilitates healing by giving you breathing room and mental energy to tackle your PTSD.

Tool Application

1. Positive distraction, as the name suggests, involves two things: 1) it needs to be something positive that is good for you and will bring you no harm, 2) and it needs to be able to distract you from your unwanted thoughts and feelings. Positive distraction activities will vary from person to person depending on their interests.

2. Positive distraction must be a means to an end meaning that it is done to give you a mental and emotional break so that you have the energy to follow it up with more direct coping skills. You must be careful not to let positive distraction become an end unto itself.

3. Some positive distraction skills you can use are listed below, but you know yourself best and what interests you:

   • Read an interesting book or watch a movie.

   • Spend time engaging in conversations with a friend, family member, or new acquaintance.

   • Do challenging games that require a lot of concentration such as Sudoku, crossword puzzles, or board games.

   • Develop an exercise routine, particularly an aerobic one such as jogging or walking.

   • Do a project around the house or apartment such as building something or making some improvement.

   • Go out shopping, even if it is just to look.

   • Pray regularly

   • Think of many other distracting activities that appeal to you that will give you a temporary break from your PTSD symptoms.

Tool 20

Cope With Panic Attacks

Many veterans report that they struggle with panic attacks. Panic attacks are a result of anxiety, but not everyone who has anxiety has panic attacks. Common symptoms experienced when having a panic attack include:

- Fast, pounding heart beat
- Flushing and sweating
- Trembling
- Dizziness
- Difficulty catching your breath
- Feeling as if you are losing your mind
- Having a strong desire to flee where you are
- Feeling a remote sensation, as if removed from your body

Panic in itself is a normal physical response to danger, similar to the fight or flight response. It can be useful if you are actually in a dangerous situation and need to respond by confronting the situation or by fleeing. Panic attacks, however, are a problem if you are not in a dangerous situation but your thoughts convince you that you are and then you have a panic attack. These panic attacks can be debilitating and create problems in your day-to-day life.

Tool Application

There are a number of different things you can do to help better cope with panic attacks. The common factor in most of them is to help you calm yourself mentally and emotionally to the point you have your panic and anxiety under control.

1. First, remind yourself that a panic attack is ultimately harmless. It basically involves a release of chemicals, such as adrenalin, into the bloodstream due to some perceived threat that causes the intense feelings. These heightened feelings will eventually pass as the chemicals are reabsorbed out of the blood.

2. An effective initial response to a panic attack is to start taking deep slow breaths making sure you are inhaling and exhaling long and slow. Some find it more helpful to inhale through the nose and slowly let the air out through the mouth. This will help to slow your heartbeat, which causes the rest of the body to relax.

3. It can also be helpful to close your eyes while you are deep breathing and imagine your self in a quiet, peaceful place, such as on the beach or beside a gently flowing stream. It is difficult for the mind to have both the panicky thoughts and to imagine being in a peaceful place. By imagining yourself in a peaceful place you will help to displace the panicky thoughts.

4. Once you have calmed down your anxiety level using the previous suggestions, you may find it helpful to involve yourself in some activity that helps to distract you away from whatever you were thinking about. For example, starting a casual conversation with someone near you, begin reading a book, listening to a MP3 player, or doing a crossword puzzle. Some people find it helpful to go over

memorized thoughts in their mind such as practicing favorite Bible verses or recalling a favorite memory.

5. Ultimately, to gain control of your panic you have to convince and remind yourself that certain situations that might cause panic, such as driving down a road or being in a crowded place, are not dangerous. Avoiding such situations typically does not help to gain better control over your panic, they only prolong it.

6. There are many good resources that go deeper into coping with panic that can be found it bookstore, libraries, and online. Take time to research these. A counselor can also teach you helpful coping skills.

The Long View

The day was growing late as Corporal Jackson and his Marine unit along with about eighty-five South Vietnamese militia entered the deserted village. Two months ago they had been through this same village and it was a bustling hive of activity of local villagers. But this time it was stone quite without anyone to be seen. Nevertheless, Jackson had an uneasy feeling they were being watched. The company commander ordered a perimeter set up and rotating shifts of sleep scheduled for the night. The men dug in deep because experience had taught them the enemy could strike hard and strike quick. Jackson was on the first shift to man the perimeter and by 2300 he was relieved. Curling up in an interior perimeter foxhole he settled down and soon drifted uneasily into a restless sleep.

The jarring explosion of incoming mortars shook Jackson from his sleep and he immediately reached for his rifle. Jumping out of the foxhole he ran back to his spot on the main perimeter. Heavy return fire was outgoing from the Marine's positions, and Jackson scanned in the darkness to see if he could identify a target. Suddenly, materializing out of the dark, a group of seven Vietcong rushed his position. He and the other two Marines in the foxhole fired and took out two of the enemy. But the other five continued their headlong rush up to the Marines. Firing down at Jackson and the other two Marines they killed one Marine before three of the enemy jumped in the foxhole. Jackson had not had time to mount his bayonet, so throwing down his weapon and drawing the knife he began to fight hand-to-hand. Immediately killing one of the enemy, he took a knife in the back shoulder from another while the other Marine fought for his life as well. Jackson turned and fell into the bottom of the foxhole as he wrestled to get the advantage from the Vietcong. Finally, he managed to dispatch the smaller man as the other Marine finished off his adversary. The other two Vietcong had already fled by the time Jackson had ended the life of his attacker. Twice more that evening the enemy attempted to overrun the Marines and South Vietnamese and twice more Jackson found himself in hand-to-hand combat. He took another wound to the leg, but the perimeter held and by daylight the enemy had been driven off for good.

Forty years later, Jackson still had moments that he struggled with his experiences in Vietnam. The struggle, however, wasn't nearly as intense now and the memories more distant. Still he had good days and bad days. He regretted he had put his family through such a hard time over the years. His three boys and daughter were now grown and on their own, but he recalled he had been very hard on them and distant. His wife remained by his side all these years and he couldn't understand why she had stayed. The early years had been the roughest, when his PTSD symptoms were the most intense. He had been so angry and cold to those around him. Flashbacks and a sense that death was always just around the next corner kept him hyper-alert and on edge. These too, however, had subsided and did not afflict him as much now.

About ten years ago, he had finally decided to seek treatment for his PTSD and he found a counselor who was very understanding and helpful. He also did a lot of reading on his own and learned alot about PTSD and actions he could take to better his life. His relationships with his children had improved, and he was thoroughly enjoying spending time with his grandchildren. He felt much more relaxed and found the simple things in life most pleasurable. He and his wife had even begun to do some traveling together in a camper they bought and their relationship was never better. His experiences and the resulting PTSD had made life a struggle, but he had made some good choices about getting help and now life was better than it had ever been.

About the Author

Ramsey Coutta is a Chaplain in the US Army and a veteran having served in Operation Iraqi Freedom. He received his Master of Divinity and PhD in Psychology from New Orleans Baptist Theological Seminary. He is a member of the National Board of Certified Counselors and has counseled extensively both privately and in the military. He and his family live near Hattiesburg, MS.